To Rachel

Before Them Set Thy Holy Will

Iconography and Pastoral Care of Those With Mental Illness

Every Blessing

Graham Reeves

Graham Reeves.

Published by

MELROSE BOOKS

An Imprint of Melrose Press Limited
St Thomas Place, Ely
Cambridgeshire
CB7 4GG, UK
www.melrosebooks.com

FIRST EDITION

Copyright © Graham Reeves 2011

The Author asserts his moral right to
be identified as the author of this work

Cover designed by Jeremy Kay

ISBN 978 1 907732 32 4

Printed and bound in Great Britain by:
CPI Group (UK) Ltd, Croydon, CR0 4YY

FSC
www.fsc.org
MIX
Paper from
responsible sources
FSC® C013604

Dedicated to the memory of
A.E.R.

Contents

Acknowledgements

This small book was never planned; it just 'happened' as a result of several things coming together at the right time. However, it would still be an array of scribbled notes, talks, and a box file of interesting resource material if it had not been for a number of encouraging people. Firstly my thanks must go to the Revd Clive Ashley, who taught me over a number of years through his actions and words the pastoral qualities of a priest working in mental health. For his constant encouragement and constructive comments on this book I thank my good friend John Wetherell. In particular I thank Fr Frank Smith. I have learned so much over the years from Fr Frank. He keeps me thinking and enables me to see things that I would never see by myself. There are echoes in the following pages of many of our conversations, for which I am greatly thankful. The Benedictine community of Alton Abbey are also deserving of thanks, especially for welcoming me as one of the family. Thanks are also due to Abbot William Hughes OSB and Dom Anselm Shobrook OSB for reading the draft manuscript and being generous in their comments. Being an avid reader I am sure many good theological writers have formed my way of thinking over the years and so in some ways have all helped to put this work together. However, any mistakes, or if I have neglected to give credit to someone, then that is my own fault and nobody else's. Of course it is right and proper to acknowledge the many patients that I meet and give my thanks to them as we journey together with Christ. Finally, I am most grateful to my wife Jackie, who not only cares for people herself in the most critical of settings, but still finds time to dig me out of a hole when I am in one, and encourages me daily. Much love to you. I must not forget my son Alex. Thank you, Alex, for the fun and laughs and for keeping the boy within me alive and active!

Foreword

Our lives are shaped by stories, stories which we tell ourselves, stories told to us by others, stories about our past, present and future. Stories frame the way we see life. As a priest and chaplain to the mentally ill, Fr Graham is sensitive to the pressing need for stories of hope in today's world and he shows us where to find them. Within the narrative of the prevailing culture, however, all we have to look forward to is an ever-increasingly vain, crazed and desperate pursuit of ways of holding the failing system together, with the concomitant manic increase in coercion and control this will entail.

Father Graham shows us how the narrative of scripture, re-presented in Orthodox iconography, confronts us with a way of picturing and seeing things that challenges the comfortable, familiar, yet destructive standards, norms and values of the consumerist world around us. Cultures given to the pursuit of selfish ends, which stand in contradistinction to those of the kingdom of God, tend to be pervaded by the exercise of an escalating demoniacal power which increasingly dehumanises and alienates people. The victims of this culture of death and destruction are hidden from view, as is anything that might threaten or undermine the, always uneasy, equilibrium of the status quo. The victims have to be disguised or hidden so that they cannot give the lie to the propaganda of the success and beneficence of the system.

From the perspective of the kingdom and the narrative of scripture, all people are seen as our neighbours and valued as those made in the image and likeness of God. Thus the good news of God's kingdom presents a radical and unpalatable challenge to cultures, built on greed and the lust for power, that treat people's lives like disposable gambling chips in some ruthless game of profit and loss. The scriptures, and the visual script of iconography, help us to become aware of, and reflect upon, another way of imagining and seeing to that propagated by those in power. This alternative vision is liberating and leads to health and wholeness and offers hope to those who, at every turn, are exposed to the malevolent abuse of a culture whose ethos and values are in violent opposition to those of scriptural narrative.

The powerful elite in any culture weave a narrative by which they seek to nurture, form and shape a society which will serve their need to retain and further develop their privileged position. Because the stories they manufacture are vital to the survival of the systems that create and maintain their status, wealth and power, they use all the means at their disposal to persuade us of the veracity of their scripts. But their story, born of greed and self-interest, is always a fabrication of lies and deceit. It is a destructive story, even for those who wield power, and this insidious narrative spreads its malevolent influence through all areas of our lives, blighting our socio-economic and political communities, private corporations, public institutions, the neighbourhoods where we live, and even adversely affecting our closest relationships. Even though their story is dressed up and presented as unchanging truth and the only way for us to live, this narrative is one of death, destruction and despair and one doomed to failure; it cannot hold together, for its foundations, built on lies and deception, are inherently fatally flawed.

But there is another story – the story of the baptised. It is a story of life, creativity and hope and it is built on truth. This latter narrative is one which the community of the baptised, are called to be immersed in. It is the story of faith, hope and love – a subversive story, one which holds out another version of reality to the one manufactured and maintained by the powerful ruling elite. It is a narrative that those in power do well to tame and domesticate because it is a report that they do not want heard, for its word, its voice, signals their demise, with their fall celebrated in the songs of the alternative community:

> *He has shown might with his arm,*
> *dispersed the arrogant of mind and heart.*
> *He has thrown down the rulers from their*
> *thrones*
> *but lifted up the lowly.*
> *The hungry he has filled with good things;*
> *the rich he has sent away empty.*
> (Luke 1: 51–53)

Songs like these, resounding throughout scripture, rejoice in a narrative of wisdom, truth and neighbourliness that runs counter to the foolishness and deceit of a culture driven by greed and self-interest, especially that of a powerful and wealthy minority, and because this alternative story has firm foundations, rooted in the truth, it is capable of standing against and triumphing over the might of empires.

The Christian community, faithful to this redemptive and salvific narrative, offers hope to those around them of another way, of a reality radically different to the one, claimed to be the only way, by those in power. This subversive and counter-cultural alternative is based upon the transcendent and invincible power of God, not upon human power and manipulation. Members of God's counter-culture, the baptised, are pleased to confess their weakness and inadequacy in the face of the demonic strength of the systems which impose themselves upon them, for it has confidence and hope in the God who is pleased to 'throw down rulers from their thrones' and 'lift up the lowly'.

Because the system, established, promoted and maintained by the ruling minority elite is based on greed and self-interest, it inevitably dehumanises and alienates all those it touches. Nevertheless we, the baptised, are tempted and coerced into colluding and collaborating with the prevailing power and are often loath to forgo the palpable degree of comfort afforded us for our consent and cooperation, especially when the alternative offered through the scriptural narrative is still future, still to be realised and, therefore, so much less tangible.

The narrative which dominates our materialist and consumerist culture exercises a powerful influence over our hearts and minds – a hold that can only be broken by a transcendent power, one which breaks in from outside.

Christ supplies such a power, which is why we, the baptised, need to soak ourselves in the story of his alternative vision of reality in order that its truth might set us free from the widely disseminated lies and illusions that possess our hearts and minds. In this way we can be true to our baptismal identity, which is essential if we are to hold out the hope of an alternative and authentic reality to a desperate and alienated world. Not only does the alternative reality of the kingdom bring hope, it also brings a joy, peace and security that the world cannot give. All this is ours if only we can hear the word of scripture and endeavour to live according to the alternative vision it presents.

This salvific vision has been faithfully captured and artistically re-presented in the wonderful script of the icon which Fr Graham helps us to explore. Fr Graham helps us to become aware of our own crises – our own moments of choice between the old and new reality – reflected in the script of the icon. In the demoniac boy we are made aware of one like ourselves, overwhelmed by powers which dehumanise and alienate him. We see the moment of choice, the present hope of another way, held out to him by Christ and we see how the boy, like us, continues to lean on, take comfort in and cling to, the old reality. Although we seek liberation in Christ we, like the demoniac, are not in our right minds, we are held captive by a world that dehumanises and alienates us and compromises our true identity. We are bound by the limitation of our imagination of what is possible. Nevertheless we are drawn to the hope of the strange future held out to us by Christ. Like the boy in the icon, we are unable to free ourselves from the overwhelming demonic forces that possess us. Our only hope is to rely on a future that comes from beyond our control, from outside all that we have known as reality. In the community of the baptised, we can reflect upon and discern together, in the light of the redemptive narrative revealed in scripture and iconography, the ways in which we have been compromised by systems of deceit and destruction, and how we might move forward together along the path of truth, liberty and holiness.

Moments of truth like these, when there is an awareness of our ambivalence and double-mindedness, create room for the Holy Spirit to work in us and do what we cannot do. Being true about our relationship with the culture of death around us, the pain and anguish it brings and about our faith and hope in Christ and his alternative future, is the way to liberation. Reflection on the narrative of scripture, and this script as it appears in the icon explored below, opens up our imagination to the possibility of such an alternative reality.

Fr Graham's insights show us how an icon can hold a mirror up to our nature and invite from us a response – challenging us to align our lives more faithfully with the truth which confronts us. The icon invites us to use our imagination to explore the scriptural narrative which, all too often, has become domesticated and tamed – rendered harmless, so that it lacks the energy necessary to move us to rise up and challenge the enervating values and norms of the surrounding secular culture that we have carelessly adopted or to which we have unwittingly succumbed. Our imaginative engagement with the text of the icon promotes an inner dialogue which leads us to explore where we fit into the picture. This, in turn, promotes a crisis wherein we are invited to opt for or against the kingdom. That such an option is possible is a cause of hope, for we not only realise that the status quo is not the only way but, also, we become aware of the beneficent alternative of another way, the way of Christ and the kingdom, which, of necessity, breaks in from beyond, transcending all human power and control.

The dominant culture, however, is hostile towards a God who is beyond our manipulation and control – a God who has radical freedom and who inspires hope and imagined alternative futures. Those who hold sway prefer a god who has been tamed, domesticated and is under their control – one who legitimises and blesses the status quo – but this is not the God of the scriptural narrative. As Fr Graham reminds us, spirituality conjured up by members of some bureaucratically assigned department, no matter how well intentioned, can only be acting on behalf of a god of their own making; it cannot be in the service of the true God. Thankfully, God is free of our control and refuses to be manipulated, even by those who set themselves up as professional spiritual practitioners. It is only because he is beyond our control that he is free to offer us the hope of an alternative to the prevailing secularism and materialism of the West. A spirituality that is subject to our control and manipulation is fit merely to serve up more of the same and thereby rob us of hope.

I am grateful to Fr Graham's insights, which help us to see that we must hold fast to that hope contained in the narrative of scripture and faithful iconography wherein we find revealed the redemptive alternative reality in which we discover our true identity and liberty as the community of the baptised. We are indebted to him for showing us how an encounter with the biblical script of an icon can be an energizing experience with the potential to awaken our imagination to the new possibilities held out to us by the good news of the kingdom and to the loving invitation to live and act in accordance with this new vision.

Frank J Smith

Introduction

People need reminding more often than
they need to be instructed.

Dr Johnson

Contained in the pages that follow is a 'reminder' –
a reminder that in our communities, congregations and
specialist units there are ordinary people who temporarily,
and in some cases with a degree of longevity, suffer from
some form of mental illness.

There is also a reminder that for the most part these same
people fail to register on the church's 'radar' and are therefore denied the many opportunities to be valued as those
beloved of Christ. I also attempt to remind all concerned,
and chaplains working in mental health in particular, that
when we look to our brothers and sisters with eyes of faith,
we are in the presence of Christ, in whose image and likeness we are all made. We are, in that sense, all 'living icons',
and it is iconography – those statements of the deepest truths
of our faith that are made visible through paint – and prayer
and right belief, that forms the benchmark for reminding us
all, not only of the task set before us, but that Christ stands
mysteriously in all human life. So, with that said, this is not
an 'instruction' book, or a 'How to …' book, or a 'self-help'

book. It simply reads as a short book, an extended reflection, of the thoughts of one who no longer wants to see Christ marginalised in the mentally ill, either individually or corporately.

These pages begin with a brief description of how the use of iconography first became a common feature of what were fairly routine talks to interested parties on chaplaincy and mental health care. This is followed by a critique of the turn towards a post-religious culture as it is experienced by the Christian chaplain in a healthcare setting of mental health. It argues for the importance of the faith-specific chaplain to remain firm, and build upon that very same faith that incorporates all of God's people in whatever state of relatedness they may be to him. Central to the argument is a theology of the icon, as it reminds us of our true identity of being in the image of God, particularly when the predominant culture seems eager to eradicate, even destroy, that image.

This book then reflects on the icon's ability, as a faithful theological statement in colour, to show the observer how slim the dividing wall is between the visible world and divine world of God's kingdom. This assures us of the nearness of God, exposing us to grace that comes from that nearness. In the light of that grace we can be confirmed as living icons regardless of how much God's image is buried.

From the position of being 'looked at' by the icon, there is a small section on hope – a hope that is experienced by both carer and cared for, diminishing that gap which sometimes exists between people in such a relationship. Not just a hope for the future, but a realised hope as the icon signifies hope for the here and now.

The second section of this small book takes a look at the icon of the demon-possessed boy (Matt. 17: 14–21; Mark 9: 14–29; Luke 9: 37–43). This detailed look is offered as a means of deepening our understanding and our mindfulness of the events surrounding the meeting of God in Christ with the brokenness not only of the boy, but with all those within the boy's circle who are also affected i.e. the father (family and carers), society (the crowd), and the disciples (the church/chaplain). It is my hope that in the end, the picture that I present in word and image may allow the reader – the observer – a clarity of vision into the calling that we all have by one degree or another, as faith communities, individuals and mental health chaplains, towards an often neglected and misunderstood area of care towards one in four of our neighbours.

Chapter 1
WORD AND ICON

I hear, and I forget. I see, and I remember.
I do, and I understand.

Ancient proverb

Professor Stephen Pattison of Cardiff University describes chaplaincy as a "liminal activity" that "takes place on the edge of religious communities" (Pattison, 2009). Even the context of chaplaincy, he adds, "occurs … on the edge of society where very particular activities are undertaken". Chaplains and chaplaincies, as part of the church's mission, can face disadvantages if they remove themselves from the faith communities of which they are part, but they can be a great advantage to the wider church when "the experience of chaplaincy tests the limits of religious concern and responsibility". Bringing the needs of others that are not always recognised beyond the boundaries of faith communities can be an important task to chaplains working on the fringes. Mental health chaplaincy is just one sphere of marginal activity, one story of the church's engagement. It is in the telling of the story, and the various engagements that chaplains are invited to, that the best opportunity arises to bring this wider context of the church's ministry to the parochial setting. In the presentation of this specific story there are the characters that weave their own individual stories as they move in and out of the picture. There are touches of humour, and moments of struggle and sadness. In some places there are even statistics and some technical jargon. However, this particular 'parochial story' only finds significance when it is told as part of a greater story, *the* story – that of the gospel of Jesus Christ, which aims to give the collection of facts and anecdotes a meaning.

More than that, by placing the life, death, and resurrection at the heart of the discussion, it no longer becomes just *my* story; it now becomes *our* story, where attitudes are changed, hearts are examined, and hopefully dialogue becomes action. Put simply, the gospel tells of God, who through the life and ministry of Christ, shows that no one is beyond His love, especially those whom society deemed untouchable, despised, and subhuman, and particularly those whose illness brought them within the orbit of mental chaos.

In these talks, attention is often given to those passages of scripture where Jesus confronts those who are categorised as demon-possessed – those whose illness results in severe mental torment. However, a word of caution at this point: it needs to be made quite clear that drawing on these scriptural accounts does not in any way assume that mental illness is due to demon possession. This is an extremely dangerous diagnostic leap to make and a subject that requires a study all to itself. Jesus and His disciples lived in a world where the existence of evil spirits was accepted, and were seen as the cause of much disturbing behaviour of the psychological kind. Opinion on this matter differs across the spectrum of Christian thought and practice; and for the purpose of this reflection, the position is adopted of demythologising the principal text being discussed because it speaks of the more common incidents of mental illness as a psychological phenomenon rather than the very rare 'demon possession' kind. For a more detailed discussion it is worth referring to the Church of England's report *A Time to Heal*, and the chapter entitled 'Deliverance from Evil' (The Archbishops' Council, 2000 p. 167. See also Appendix 1).

The aim of drawing these scriptural episodes into the story is to show quite categorically that Christ had a special concern for those separated and marginalised due to mental distress. Contributing factors to Christ's attitude may have been the occasions when He himself faced accusations of the scribes and Pharisees of being possessed, and His own family suggesting that He was out of His mind (Matt. 12: 22–29; Mark 3: 22–27; Luke 11: 14–22). This may have been something that Christ confronted on a regular basis. For example, the synoptic gospels place healing as evidence that in Christ, the Kingdom of God was now breaking in. In the Gospels of Mark and Luke the first act of healing is of the man in the synagogue, who was described as having an evil spirit. To come to a conclusion as to whether this was a case of demon possession (and therefore providing the initial theological link towards the authority of Jesus and His control over Satan's household), or a culturally conditioned way of expressing an explanation for a form of mental illness, will depend on one's own personal understanding and theological/ecclesiological formation. Within this context it serves the purpose of showing that mental distress, and Christ's encounter with it, appears high on the Gospel agenda.

The most useable example I have found for these discussions is the account of the healing of the demon-possessed boy (or the boy with epilepsy, as some translations refer to it), in Matt. 17: 14–21; Mark 9: 14–19; and Luke 9: 37–43. It has become the most useable for three reasons. (There was eventually to be a fourth reason, which will be explored more fully later.)

Reason 1. The passage in the synoptics confirms that Christ was passionate about engaging, bringing hope and new life to those who suffered with mental illness. Therefore it can be argued that the importance given to this aspect of ministry by Christ should be equally as important to the church.

Reason 2. The language employed by Matthew. The boy is described by the Greek word *seleniazomai*, which means 'moonstruck'. Translated into the vernacular, it sometimes appears literally as 'lunatic' e.g. in the KJV (King James Version). Unfortunately, this is the kind of language that people use and immediately understand. So by highlighting this there is an instant verbal engagement with the 'parochial' personal story and the larger Gospel story.

Reason 3. Again, a verbal connection. The Greek of Matthew's text gives an indication of the torment of those with mental illness, which was recognised by the author as being something very close to the personal suffering of Christ himself. This is what John Nolland says about the language used by Matthew in verse 17:

> *With one exception, Matthew uses kakos (lit. 'badly') exclusively with reference to the sufferings of those cured by Jesus. The idiom is normally kakos ekein (lit. 'have badly'), but here it is the stronger kakos pasxien ('suffer badly') using a verb normally reserved for the sufferings of Jesus.*
>
> Nolland (2005, p. 711)

What Matthew seems to be saying is that those who suffer and manifest mental torment – those who are 'demonised' – have a particular 'Christ likeness' about them. There seems to be a strong empathy with this kind of human suffering.

Every work related talk given would result in the standard address based around this particular Gospel reading, supplemented with details from the same account in both Mark and Luke – a sort of exegesis weaved around lived and ongoing experience, inviting the listeners to think about the importance of participating in this story within their own particular context, be it parish or community group. However, being mindful of the human capacity to be overwhelmed by words triggered a memory of something heard many years ago. It went something like "The Word became flesh and dwelt amongst us, and sometimes all we do is turn that reality back into words". It was then that the opportunity presented itself to draw upon the use of iconography, an important part of my own faith and formation, to 'incarnate' each talk.

While pondering this possibility, I discovered the fourteenth-century Orthodox icon, from a monastery in Serbia, of the very text I used in the talks: *The Healing of the Demon-Possessed Boy*. Introducing the icon into the talks gave me the fourth reason for using this particular text in its synoptic variations. For then a deeper meaning could be seen that the text alone could not easily produce.

The possibility of bringing sacred text and icon together became a type of Emmaus Road experience (Luke 24: 13–32). The personal stories of the disciples as they travelled, full of sadness and questions, is transformed by the hidden presence of the risen Christ as He places their experience into the bigger story of God's salvific plan. In this dialogue the process of understanding and recognition begins to take place, for their hearts burned within them. But it is not until they sit down and witness Christ breaking bread that the full realisation of the words takes place. It is in the 'seeing' of the event that makes the 'hearing' fully comprehensible. This link between hearing and seeing is well demonstrated in the theology of iconography. Michael Quenot writes:

> ... *how much do we really understand about the impact of the visual on our hearing and, reciprocally, of hearing on our sight? The subject is of prime importance when we re-*

> *call that in Orthodoxy, the word of God in*
> *the sacred scriptures, our liturgical texts*
> *and icons are all intimately linked togeth-*
> *er... The word of God has in the icon an ir-*
> *replaceable support, because the icon offers*
> *a more vivid revelation of the mystery that*
> *the word proclaims... Modern science con-*
> *firms that what we hear results from what*
> *we see.*

Quenot (1991a, p. 119)

For the most part, particularly in the West, faith is expressed, and theology learned and explored, primarily through words, both oral and written. That is hardly surprising since our principal source for discovering and understanding God's relation with His creation is through the Bible. Everything comes back to our foundation document – the place where God is revealed, His ways are discerned, and our salvation is worked out. The icon does no less. The Gospel proclaims in words the story of humanity's salvation. The icon proclaims visually, in colour and form, the same story. Fr Steven Bigham explains this very clearly:

> *Just as words and concepts can paint a ra-*
> *tional image of the mystery of salvation, a*
> *printed image can also show the salvation*
> *experience. In the same as words, colors*
> *can paint the same mystery in a visual im-*
> *age, and both mediums of expression must*

> *be faithful to the church's experience. Ico-*
> *nography is therefore a theological art be-*
> *cause it expresses, represents, makes vis-*
> *ible, in forms and colors, the same content*
> *that is expressed in written documents.*
>
> Bigham (1998, p. 44)

And a little further he adds, "Theologians of the image are therefore just as important as theologians of the word."

Our words, our actions, what we say and what we do (the church's experience), must be the product of right belief – a belief formed, shaped and practised by scripture, tradition, councils, creeds and liturgy; and formed by examining the lives of countless holy men and women who, through the ages, and in our present day, make Christ known. The icons are products of this right belief and can be seen as true statements of the church's teaching and practice. Equally, when the icon 'looks back' at us, when our eyes take in the themes, the forms and the colours, the experience that it conveys and, is faithful to, invites and reminds us that this is what *we* must be faithful to and make known through our individual and corporate experience.

The church's message is contained in the image. The image gazes back on the church, reminding her of what that message is. In the case of the icon of the demon-possessed boy, we see a true and faithful statement of the church's experience brought into visual form. Confronting this visual form liturgically, prayerfully, meditatively, and didactically, can act as a vehicle for translating the theology of the icon, taking the visual form back into practice and experience. This can be both uncomfortable for communities and individuals that neglect this aspect of the church's experience and practice, and it can be transforming and liberating to those that suffer, to see their experience of isolation transformed into acceptance, marginalisation into inclusion, misunderstanding into understanding, and fragmentation into growth towards wholeness – in effect, the journey from darkness to light. This journey is itself grounded in the technique used to 'write' an icon. The application of the paint begins with the dark colours, eventually leading to the lighter colours, literally bringing light out of darkness. What the iconographer accomplishes, pastoral care aims to accomplish with the 'living icons' in our care: working gently towards the light of healing from the darkness of illness.

With the introduction of the icon into the pastoral encounter, a whole new world of possibilities for meaning, understanding and engagement are revealed, not only into the lives of those who suffer, but also to recall faith-specific healthcare chaplaincy back to its theological roots, including the church, who cannot afford to neglect this valuable group of people. Valuable because they are God's and valuable because Christ defied all the cultural tendencies of His time – tendencies that were aimed at denying these sufferers life and bringing them into His company.

Within the healthcare setting, Christian chaplains are having to renegotiate their position in a world where post-religious spiritualities are claiming much more prominence as a means for seeking meaning. These are spiritualities usually devoid of any discernable structure or base other than the problematic 'stand alone' or 'pick and mix' kind. It is into this complicated mix that, with discernment and care and gentleness, the icon can help to provide a firm foundation for us to rediscover our identities in relation to God, and function as channels of God's desire to reach out and welcome. The integrating of iconography into pastoral care has opened up another way for us to be able to be reminded that the image of God is to be seen and encountered in every human being, even when one has to look very deeply. Also, the joy of seeing others catch a glimpse of that for themselves when they are in the darkest of places and in the most meaningless of situations, is very rewarding.

Chapter 2
RECLAIMING OUR TRUE IDENTITY

They drew a circle that shut me out
Heretic, rebel, a thing to flout,
But love and I had the wit to win,
We drew a circle that took them in.
Nineteenth-century American poet

There is in our culture a new era of iconoclasm. By that I do not mean the literal, wilful destruction of iconography reminiscent of the eighth- and ninth-century Byzantium period. I am thinking more of a culture that is gradually erasing from humanity the fundamental theological truth that we are made in the image and likeness of God, and are in fact living icons. Within the context of pastoral care, what is the basis for making such a claim? Firstly, this chapter will identify features of the iconoclasts that provide the basis for the argument, and then it will go on to apply these criteria within the contemporary debate that surrounds the provision of spiritual and religious care in the context of the healthcare setting. While focusing specifically on the experience of chaplaincy, the following argument is just as relevant for church communities, for the chaplain is on the front line of mission and ministry and can have much to say to the church as it, too, engages with its host culture.

The iconoclast controversy of the eighth and ninth centuries in the Byzantine period had a number of causes. Primarily the conflict lay in the nature of the divine and whether it was possible to represent God, Christ, the Holy Mother and the saints in an artistic form. On another level the argument raised questions about matter, about whether God, through the incarnation of Christ, made holy the whole created order and everything within it. In an essay about the iconoclastic controversy, Peter Brown writes:

> *The iconoclast controversy was a debate on the position of the holy in Byzantine society. On the issue of what was holy and what was not, the iconoclasts were firm and unambiguous. Certain material objects were holy because they had been solemnly blessed by ordained priests ... Icons could not be holy because they had received no consecration from above.*
>
> Brown (1973, pp. 5–6)

Reflecting on this point, Kallistos Ware in his contribution towards a series of edited essays by Harries, Mayr-Harting adds:

> *Among the questions raised by the contro-*
> *versy were these: Who controls the holy?*
> *How far should the divine be allowed to im-*
> *pinge upon the human world? Can the holy*
> *be narrowly restricted? ... Or does it spill*
> *out more unpredictably – we might even say,*
> *more untidily – into every aspect of human*
> *life?*
>
> Harries, Mayr-Harting (2001a, p. 91)

For the iconoclasts, the influence of the divine was to be restricted

> *... to specific areas where the clergy were in*
> *full control, such as the Eucharist; and they*
> *argued that icons could not be holy because*
> *no specific prayer of blessing had been said*
> *over them.*
>
> Harries, Mayr-Harting (2001b, p. 92)

However, the iconophiles did not subscribe to this at all. It was their belief that

> *... no specific human initiative is needed in*
> *order to bring something into the realm of*
> *the holy, for all that God has created is by its*
> *very nature intrinsically sacred. The whole*
> *world is a sacrament of the divine presence,*
> *the realm of matter in its entirety ...*

Harries, Mayr-Harting (2001b, p. 92)

To put it in very simplistic terms, the iconoclasts set a boundary around God, limiting His presence to specific roles and functions of those called by the church through ordination. In refusing to accept that icons are bearers of the holiness of God, they were also refusing to accept that through the incarnation, of God taking on flesh, taking on human matter, the whole of the created order also reflected the glory of God. Matter was not to be despised; it was not to be placed beyond the realms of what was holy.

God's creation, as described by the book Genesis, is "very good". Choosing to take upon Himself human flesh, created flesh, endorses this goodness. Not just flesh, but the whole creation. Rowan Williams writes:

> ... because God's creation is wider than the human race, what is true of humans is also true of things. The Greek theologians of the early church sometimes spoke of each element in the material world carrying a 'word' from God, revealing an aspect of God's life and wisdom.

Williams (2007a, p. 5)

To disbelieve this, which it seems the iconoclasts were doing, was to deny the universality and greatness of God. To believe this, as the iconophiles did, was to see that "God has 'deified' matter, making it 'spirit bearing'; and if flesh has become a vehicle of the spirit, then so, though in a different way, can wood and paint" (Ware, 1997, p. 33).

So we are presented within the history of a particular culture the ideas and theology of a group with a view to initiate change in the most destructive of ways, that not only aimed to bring about the limitation of God, but also the limitation of His creation. For the faith-specific chaplain (Christian) working in healthcare at the beginning of the twenty-first century, the parallels that exist between this particular feature of the iconoclastic controversy and the practice and policies of post-modern chaplaincy (or spiritual care departments, as most like to be called now) are very familiar indeed.

Every age has a particular way of looking at the world and at the human response to the world. We find ourselves at this moment in our history living through what has commonly been called 'post-modernity'. This is much too big a subject to go into in any depth here, but for the purpose of this argument the rise in spirituality, as opposed to religion, is a characteristic of a post-modern culture.

To give a flavour of what this means I have selected a few quotations, from within and outside of the healthcare setting, to present the post-modern picture of spirituality and religion. Bishop Tom Wright, in his usual clear and insightful way writes:

> *Within post-modernity, God is sometimes assumed to be a very old silly dream that's long gone, but equally within the New Age*

movement there are gods of all sorts, gods aplenty, coming bubbling up at us from all corners, and not necessarily the Christian God by any manner of means. Everyone now wants spirituality, but ironically they don't think, in fact most of them don't think, that you can find it in the church.

Wright (2005)

With a little more detail, Sandra M. Schneider IHM writes:

...post-modernity fosters the pursuit of idiosyncratic and non-religious spirituality ... characterised by fragmentation of thought and experience which focuses attention on the present moment, an immediate satisfaction, in what works for me ... A non-religious spirituality makes no distinct claims, imposes no moral authority outside one's own conscience, creates no necessary personal relationships or social responsibilities and can be changed or abandoned whenever it seems to work for the practitioner ... Clearly such a spirituality is much more compatible with a post-modern sensibility than the religion of any church, especially Christianity.

Schneider (2000a, pp. 11–12)

So, the post-modern influence on spirituality is literally: anything goes! If it feels good then stick with it. It is stand-alone and no longer needs to be attached to the outdated, over-demanding, exclusive and even damaging religion that spirituality was once associated with (and there are periods during the church's history, and in certain individuals, where this is true, but there is such a thing as 'good religion'). John Swinton writes:

> *The migration of spirituality from the religious to the secular has led to a change in the meaning of spirituality as popularly conceived. Rather than being viewed as a specifically religious concept, spirituality has broadened its meaning into a more diffuse human need that can be met quite apart from institutionalised religious structures.*
>
> Swinton (2001, p. 11)

This splitting away of the spiritual from the religious is presented in John Swinton's book in a diagrammatic form which illustrates visually the post-modern turn to spirituality and its sphere of influence, particularly for healthcare professionals including faith-specific chaplains. The diagram is a circle marked 'spirituality' and contained inside this circle is a smaller circle marked 'religion'. This demonstrates clearly the compartmentalisation of religion, ring-fencing religion, if you like, from the wider experience of post-modern spirituality.

On one level this 'spirituality removed from religion' project needs to be applauded. Any move towards improving and finding a greater depth towards patient understanding and care needs to be embraced. However, this can create an imbalance in the healthcare setting, occasionally resulting in the marginalisation of the religious practitioner along with the religious care that is practised. However, it is my opinion that when spirituality is properly relocated within its religious foundations, faith-specific chaplaincy can once again find a strong voice and a relevance without the need to become either a 'spiritual care giver' or a 'spiritual care department'. Listen to one voice within the healthcare setting to explain what I am trying to describe.

> *Vanilla spirituality: the mistaken belief that at its very core the human person is/has an amorphous spiritual dimension; certainly for a Catholic this is only partly true. The full story is that the dimension is fundamentally Christological. To people of faith, whether Muslim, Jew or Christian, it is the context of belief that defines the person and gives identity. Where a secular mind might have difficulty admitting of this, it would be less challenged by the vaguely identifiable phenomenon of spirituality since it signifies both everything and nothing. Far less messy and partisan than all that troublesome religion. Changed your name to Dept. of Spiritual*

Care recently and thought nothing of it? Per-
haps I am paranoid, but it worries me.

Mason (2006, p. 66)

From a faith-specific point of view, Fr Mason's comments are pertinent, particularly seeing at the heart of humanity a Christological dimension. The role of priest and chaplain in the healthcare setting is one of 'always meet people where they are'. Timothy Radcliffe writes:

> *Wherever we are, in whatever confusions or*
> *messes we find ourselves, this is the start-*
> *ing point of our journey home ... We begin*
> *where they are now ... In whatever mess we*
> *may be living, a story can be told that will*
> *make sense of it, and a story that leads to*
> *the Kingdom.*
>
> Radcliffe (2005, p. 42)

This satisfies the regime that we are meeting spiritual needs, with or without any religious content, depending on the encounter. However, when a pastoral encounter with the 'spiritual' rather than the 'religious' occurs, the chaplain meets that person as a representative of the universal and inclusive church. In a dialogue, whether faith-specific or not, a space is created – a meeting place – where God can be experienced as welcoming, loving and accepting. Christian chaplaincy has always said "yes" to everyone that it encounters, in whatever condition the one encountered might be in. Fundamentally, that is because at the heart of every encounter, Christ dwells in the person that one is in dialogue with. As Rowan Williams writes:

> *Christianity teaches that each person is created by God with a distinct calling and capacity ... People may refuse their calling or remain stubbornly unaware of it, but God continues to call them and offer them what they need to fulfil their calling.*
>
> Williams (2007b, p. 4)

This is intrinsic to our calling by God, as Christian chaplain Edward Lewis writes:

> *Chaplains are there as authorised representatives to minister God's love and care. That will be expressed in different ways for the different denominations and faiths ... There is also a vital ministry to those who are themselves searching, whose spirituality might not be articulated through a faith, but who are fellow travellers.*
>
> Lewis (2005, p. 40)

As Anglican or Catholic chaplains, we share in the ministry of the bishop and are just as much accountable to the church as to the National Health Service (NHS). We are first called as priests, then chaplains. The statement that comes the closest to what this argument so far has been moving towards is one written by the Association of Hospice and Palliative Care Chaplaincy. It states, "Although spiritual care is not necessarily religious care, religious care, at its best, should always be spiritual" (NHS, 2003, p. 5).

In light of this, and what I have said so far, I would want to adjust John Swinton's diagram as mentioned earlier to reflect the faith-specific chaplaincy approach. Here the positions are reversed. Now, through the faith-specific approach, the faith or religious 'bit' isn't ring-fenced; it becomes the circle containing within itself a 'spirituality' element because we cannot but see everything from a Christological, and therefore an incarnational, perspective. This is the stream from which all our encounters must ultimately find meaning. In the sixth Norman Autton lecture, Jane Williams takes the Christological and the incarnational as the ground of our understanding. She says:

> ... when the health service tries to unpack what it means by spirituality ... what it usually means by that word is to do with meaning and significance, as far as I can see. But the problem is that meaning and significance can't be invented. You cannot give somebody meaning and significance simply by saying this is the meaning and significance department. They have to flow from some kind of recognisable structures, structures in which we find our place and our values and so in

which we know our meaning and our sig-
nificance. For the Christian chaplain, the
structure from which all meaning flows and
within which we know human life to be in-
finitely valuable is precisely this doctrine of
God...

Williams. J (2007, p. 5)

Bringing this back full circle to my original assertion that we are in a new era of iconoclasm, the threads of this argument can be drawn together and a counter-proposal suggested which will hopefully show that the icon can be a means of reinvigorating and introducing something fresh into the chaplain's engagement with his/her own practice and the healthcare arena. (This also applies to those in church communities.)

To engage with the human condition at a spiritual level where God either plays no part at all or is reduced to something that is made in the image of the bearer rather than the one who beholds, is to deny that person his or her uniqueness as a living icon, as someone who is due the same honour as Christ Himself. It is to gaze upon blank faces, to collude with a system that makes a person a slave to a cultural movement. The incarnation – God taking on flesh in Jesus Christ – hallows all flesh and matter. The human face of Jesus bears the invisible face of God. "Whoever has seen me has seen the Father," says Christ (John 14: 9). This is the basis by which the image of God, the Christ of God, the icon of God, can be depicted in the form of holy art which mediates the presence of God in a unique way. And when we are in the presence of an icon of Christ or His Mother or a saint or a biblical scene, we are confronted with the truth of the Gospel. And part of that truth is to realise that the beauty of God is the beauty within the one who gazes upon the icon, the one who himself/herself is a living icon.

We began with a quote from Kallistos Ware, who highlighted, via several questions, particular features of the iconoclastic argument. The questions can now be posed again. He asked, "Who controls the holy?" In a culture characterised by a post-modern shift, the holy is controlled and kept in control by those who advocate a spirituality detached from good reflective religion or a faith-specific standpoint. The holy, at worse, has become a negative to be replaced by the spirituality of our age, and at best is sectioned off for certain individuals and for specific functions.

Kallistos Ware's second question: "How far should the divine be allowed to impinge on the human world?" In the healthcare setting the policies and procedures are quite clear. The divine is allowed to impinge within the human world of faith-practising people only. The faith-specific chaplain is the only one to deliver this form of care, that is, of course, if the divine is of God and not the divine of some other larger-than-self entity.

The third question: "Can the holy be narrowly restricted, or does it spill out more unpredictably?" is the same as asking whether or not we can pin down the holy. Those who favour the turn to post-religious spiritualities detached from authentic faith-specific spirituality would argue that the holy can be pinned down, partitioned off, and in fact demand that this approach is adhered to for fear of unwelcome overt religious pushiness. For a trained healthcare chaplain this is never an issue, on the grounds of proper conduct demanded by the chaplaincy bodies, and the codes of conduct and policies of the NHS. This was mentioned earlier and as Schneider says:

> *We do not advance as onto a field of battle with our tradition as shield against heresy, or paganism or, worse yet, as a sword with which to vanquish the other. Nor, however, do we check our faith tradition at the door ... and enter as a tabula rasa. Rather we enter, undefended, securely rooted in our Christian faith tradition that we have internalised through study and practice as our own living spirituality, knowing that our truth can never be ultimately threatened by the truth of the other.*

> Schneider (2000b, p. 18)

And Kallistos Ware's final question: "Does it spill out more unpredictably?" Of course it does! The theology that makes the icon an authentic experience of God is the same theology that makes the human person an authentic experience of God. But it may be that we will need to look a little harder and a little deeper into the face of the one we are engaged with to see the image of God. The whole of creation is filled with the glory of God and that glory will spill out in the most unpredictable of ways, in the most unpredictable of people, in the most unpredictable of situations. The holy icons invite us into the certainty of this unpredictability, as we will go on to see.

Chapter 3
THE ICON AND THE NEARNESS OF GOD

Lord of the excluded,
Open my eyes to those I would prefer not to
see,
Open my life to those I would prefer not to
know,
Open my heart to those I would prefer not to
love,
And so open my eyes to see
Where I exclude you.

Iona Community

The fullness of God shines out from the face of Christ, and in being bathed in this divine light, the object of Christ's love, the one gazing into this light, is then invited to be drawn out, exposed and healed. On Mt Sinai, when Moses asked to see God he was told, "You cannot see my face, for no one shall see me and live" (Exodus 33: 20). However, this hiddenness of God is revealed, made approachable, as He takes on flesh through Christ. Now we are given an image of God that we can see, and the old prohibition is reversed, for to look on the face of God in Christ is to live.

There is a scene from the film *Patch Adams* where Patch discharges himself from the psychiatric unit in order to follow a path of helping others. In the scene the psychiatrist disputes with Patch over the nature of care, and he maintains that as the professional, care is his primary role, to which Patch replies, "But you suck at it; you don't even look at someone when they are talking to you." To gaze on the face of Christ in the icon is to be fully engaged by God. The full-face gaze and the eye contact brings the observer into an intimate closeness of full attendance. And this gaze isn't the gaze of the clinician or any other professional. Nor is it the voyeuristic half-gaze or purposeful non-gaze of a judgemental public. This is the gaze of the creator, who sees in the created well beyond the chaos, the confusion and the sin, to something that is of immense value. Aiden Hart remarks:

> *Hell is standing back to back, being deprived of other people's faces. Heaven is to behold the face of the Lord and the face of my brothers and sisters.*

Hart (2000a, p.1)

Mental illness becomes for many that place of hell where others choose not to look, to wilfully look away.

The face-to-face encounter makes God present in a way that words or talking therapies cannot. A common characteristic of the isolated patient, confused by illness, confused by a cocktail of medication, removed from what is familiar, whose faith is challenged by these circumstances, is the feeling of God's remoteness, His absence. Within the pastoral encounter assurances can be given and many theologically loaded examples can be offered through the medium of speech and word that aims to make the presence of God a reality. However, words are easily forgotten. But when this remoteness, that feeling that God is absent, is challenged by the presence of the icon, a different kind of influence other than the verbal argument is introduced. Richard Temple gives some idea of what this influence is when he writes about the "icon not made with hands":

> *An image or a portrait of a man can help exert his influence in his absence. In other words his portrait seems to remind us that he exists after he has gone ... hence the universal popularity of the photograph or the snapshot of a loved person or member of the family ...*
>
> Temple (1982, p. 10)

So the icon might work as a picture or portrait might, but remember, it is neither, and care should be taken not to reduce it to such, primarily because a picture or photograph can signify the presence of a loved one when the loved one is absent, but the icon is the signifier of the loved one who is present and, in effect, can never be absent. Therefore the icon is much more. It is a theological statement in colour, and with prayer and guidance it will inform the pastoral encounter just as much by what isn't seen as what can be seen. (More will be said on this when we come to look at and be looked at by the icon of the healing of the demon-possessed boy.)

The icon becomes a visual experience of God meeting us, drawing us into His gaze, and showing us, particularly with the festal icons of miracles and parables, and the icons of the saints, what life is like and can be like.

In a lecture given by Dr Clark Carlton and Frank Schaefer (Carlton and Schaefer), Dr Carlton, drawing on the work of Cornel West, talks about the 'normative gaze'. The normative gaze creates the ideal measure of humanity, a standard by which we judge ourselves. The normative gaze of the fashion industry, for example, is one where we should all be superthin, or have tanned six-pack bodies. In the same way, icons create a normative gaze. When we look at them, worship with them and pray with them, we see what human life should be like. This is the standard we judge ourselves by as we are drawn to that light that brightens the light within us. For the icon shows us not only how things ought to be, the standard that it sets, but it shows us how things are and will be, because this is the Kingdom we are gazing into.

And isn't this what Christ himself is doing? He looks to the Father and does only what he sees the Father doing. Whatever the Father does the Son does (John 5: 19–20). God is the foundational normative gaze, whose presence shines through the Son and the events of the icon, to rest on the gaze of the observer, presenting an alternative way of being that demands nothing more than being totally oneself.

Surrounded by icons in his hermitage chapel, Aiden Hart reflects that those who visit

... can just be, and by being, by looking ...
they meet something of God's beauty. In ex-
periencing this divine beauty through icons,
they discover something of their own dignity
as living icons of God. And this is a dignity
given rather than earned. A dignity to be re-
ceived and nurtured rather than fabricated.

Hart (2000b, p. 1)

The icon makes present the Gospel imperative of inclusion, of 'being with' rather than 'being apart' or separated. Of freedom to stand accepted and worthy of being called into communion with God and each other. This is the dignity which the icon offers, the immense gift to those in a poverty of unacceptability to others and quite often themselves. This unacceptability that is given life by the stigma attached to those with mental illness can be challenged by the careful drawing out of the worth and importance of the icons, which become just as applicable to every person as living icons. To explain, Gillian Crow writes:

... icons are a reminder that we are all im-
ages – icons – of God. When a priest censes
the church he goes around censing all the
icons in it – and also all the people – because
people are holy icons of God ... Painted icons
become covered with soot and grime with
age, sometimes to the point where the sub-
ject is barely recognisable. They can be dam-

30

> *aged, overpainted, broken; they can fall into the wrong hands and be badly treated. When this happens they are not thrown out with the rubbish but are carefully and lovingly mended and restored ... so it should be with living icons ...*
>
> Crow (2008, p. 97)

Once again, to be in the presence of the icons, to be brought into the scrutiny of them, is to be lead towards a place of affirmation. The unacceptability, the worthlessness projected and fostered by a culture that values success and beauty above everything else, all these projections from without and the fears, chaos, the turmoil from within, go towards disfiguring and blurring the beauty that lies beneath. At the very heart the true image awaits to be lovingly restored and brought to the surface. Like Aaron's blessing (Numbers 6: 24–26.) we stand in a place where the Lord's face shines upon us, bringing grace, encounter and peace. Inviting a person to see this about himself/herself is to open the possibility of seeing hope amidst constant struggle.

Chapter 4
THE ICON – A PLACE OF HOPE

When you say a situation or a person is
hopeless you are slamming the door in the
face of God.

Charles L. Allen

A priest friend once said that as a spiritual
father his aim was to give people hope, for if
people had hope, then faith and love would
follow. Perhaps therein lies the icon's power
for pastoral carers.

Hart (2000c, p. 5)

Something similar was once said by the late Bishop Morris
Maddocks, one-time advisor to the Archbishop of Canterbury
on the healing ministry. He said, "Never leave any pastoral
encounter without giving some small grain of hope." This is
sound pastoral advice, but not always easy to do, especially
in the face of mental illness, where someone is engulfed
by hopelessness. Even in those dark, seemingly hopeless
situations there is still the pastoral principle employed by
many a chaplain/carer, and that is a vicarious holding on to
hope. Marion L.S. Carson makes this point in her book *The*

Pastoral Care of People with Mental Health Problems.

> *In the face of overwhelming circumstances*
> *we may have to cling onto the idea of hope*
> *by sheer will. In severe depression, how-*
> *ever, this becomes impossible and the very*
> *concept of hope can seem at best incompre-*
> *hensible and at worst a lie. Pastoral care*
> *includes holding onto that hope on behalf*
> *of those who cannot, until they are able to*
> *rediscover it for themselves.*
>
> Carson (2008, p. 7)

However, even holding on to hope for someone else can be a lot easier said than done, as the pastoral care giver or chaplain factors in personal fatigue, the enormity of the struggle being played out before their eyes, compassion fatigue and the sense of one's own hopelessness. There is also the potential as the one who is the dispenser and keeper of hope to set up an unbalanced pastoral encounter of the cared for and the carer; the one who is whole and the one who is broken; the classic 'them' and 'us' situation. To all these varying aspects of care the icon can say something that enlarges our view of hope, which incorporates both carer/chaplain and patient as partners in the journey. As Aiden Hart puts it, this is the "power" of the icon.

Would it be presumptuous to think that all iconographers are people of hope? As people firmly rooted in the present world, they present to us through the very stuff of creation

– wood, paint etc – a future world of which we are able to come close to and make our own. These everyday organic things are employed sacramentally, so to speak; brought together through prayer, reflection and in union with the church, to bring the Kingdom before us.

Gathered before the icon of the demon-possessed boy, with all one's energies forced into a narrow focus determined by the boundaries of illness, the second part of this short book will attempt to show how the transfigured world into which we are drawn begins to transfigure those bits of ourselves that we immediately begin to associate with in the icon. The glimpse into our present/future with God is the offer of wellbeing, of a space to breathe, of new life. A place where we can be free to be ourselves as we have always been seen by God.

For the icon opens up for us not only a space *of* hope, but a space *to* hope. I wrote earlier of holding hope; the icon shows this hope of which we are speaking of. It is an expression of the hope which is at the heart of all Christian living and dying. A hope that declares and anticipates that God is with us, mysteriously, maybe untidily and seemingly fleetingly, but then wholly, fully, and for all eternity. The icon is a preventative to pushing hope somewhere, sometime in the future (which is where hope is usually situated) – something for another time other than now, especially when all the evidence and the pastoral clichés ("I will hold on to hope for you") show that the one in despair doesn't have it in the present. The embrace of the icon's presence, that which it signifies and points us towards, that which spills out before us, is a glimpse of hope for now, this moment, right where we are. In the present lie our future hopes, and our future hope floods into our present.

In scripture, God declares that He is with His people. This hope for creation and humanity never leaves the pages of scripture, culminating in the person of Christ, who is our hope enfleshed. Scripture tells us through a multitude of voices and through several different genres how this hope is brought alive. As Rowan Williams writes:

> *... the hope described in the Bible is connected not to any aspect of our lives but to God's faithful commitment to the whole of what He has made.*
>
> Williams (2007c, p. 143)

It is God who ultimately holds hope and there is no one beyond the scope of this assurance. What the icon does is show this hope visually. Scripture tells us this, and the icon shows it.

Earlier in this book, reference was made to both chaplain/carer and the patient as 'partners' in the journey. In the psychiatric setting (and in several other similar settings) there is a danger of portraying the ministry of care as just another therapy, especially when chaplains are being encouraged more and more to become professionals in an environment where there is an increase in professionalism. This can create a distinction between those who are well, whole (even holy), and those who are ill, broken and incomplete. When the culture and the person-to-person encounter sets up these roles the spectre of control isn't far away, resulting in a 'them' and 'us' relationship. Being with a fellow traveller, a partner on the journey in the presence of the icon, vastly reduces the pitfall of control and the hierarchies of wellbeing. Listen again to Aiden Hart:

> The icon can in fact abolish the dichotomy of helper and helped, or at least make the 'gap' tiny in comparison to the gap between them both and the beauty of holiness ... Realisation of this infuses a humility in the counsellor which can only rebound in the good of the counselee. They are on a journey together and the icon stands as a little jewel reflecting something of the light of the transfiguration which, if they want it, awaits them. Also, certainly for an orthodox spiritual guide and potentially for other counsellors, the icon shares the onus of caring. At its fullest this means that the icons remind the carer that the saints are working with them to meet whatever needs there are. But for those who do not believe this, simply as a visual aid the icon still remains effective as a third party, expanding the didactic relationship into a healthier triadic one.
>
> Hart (2000d, p. 4)

Sitting together in prayer, in silence, in dialogue over aspects of the icon, we do so as equals: equally loved by God, equally growing towards a greater vision and understanding of just 'being' in the presence of God, and equally being brought into the presence of a hope that is held and offered by God for each of us.

Drawing the first part of this book to a conclusion, some words of Abbot Christopher Jamison of Worth Abbey locate the importance of hope within the boundaries of faith and religion, right in the place where this essay began. He writes:

> *The key spiritual resource that religion offers is hope. "The future of humanity," the church stated at the Second Vatican Council, "lies in the hands of those able to pass on to future generations reasons for living and hoping." Reasons for living and hoping are the heart of true religion, and the greatest gift that religion gives to humanity.*
>
> Jamison (2006, p. 167)

This is the unique calling of faith-specific chaplaincy, and in terms of this essay, the Christian faith, and I hope to show in the second part of this essay how the icon of the healing of the demon-possessed boy offers many reasons "for living and hoping" – an open window by which the light of God's transcended world can pour into the lives of all of us who journey towards a place of life and hope.

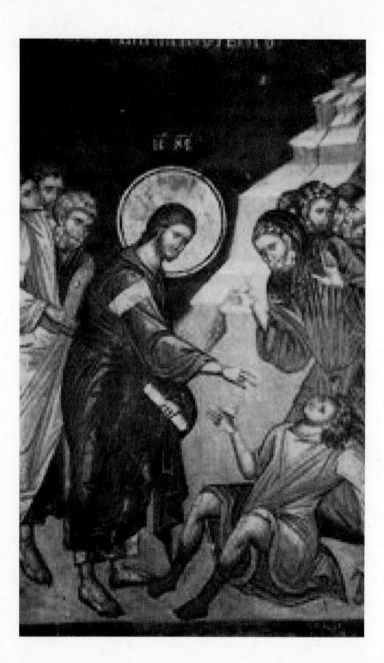

Chapter 5
THE ICON OF CHRIST HEALING
THE DEMON-POSSESSED BOY

BRIEF OVERVIEW

The icon entitled *Christ Healing the Demon-Possessed Boy*, is a deeply engaging presentation of the events that greeted Jesus and the disciples Peter, James and John as they completed their descent from the Mount of Transfiguration. As the eye takes in the scene that is made visible in form and colour from the written accounts in the synoptic gospels, there is a definite increase in activity and energy as the eye moves from left to right.

From the contemplation and concentration of Peter, James and John, the authoritative figure of Christ gives way to a scene filled with energy and movement, At Christ's feet lays the boy, contorted, disorientated and dwarfed by all around. Behind the boy stands his father, hands raised in exasperation and frustration; and behind him again, the crowd, consisting of the remaining disciples and teachers of the law, who are too preoccupied with argumentative discourse to notice the moment of healing.

To scan the icon we can experience this movement

from calm to chaos. However, to be more correct in our contemplation of the icon, the iconographer correctly places Christ, using the convention of hierarchical perspective, as our primary focus. Now as our eyes move out from Christ, we see the scene as one of calm *behind* Him, and action and chaos in *front* of Him. We need to bear this in mind in our contemplation of the icon, for it provides a sound theological framework for all that is happening in the scene, and for all that we will go on to do as we are transformed by it.

The following reflections are a result of many hours spent in its presence, and many hours integrating the influence it has had into pastoral encounters with the living icons that share the world of mental illness.

The Figure of Christ

Compared with the other figures in the icon Christ is the largest figure, denoting His importance, and our eyes are immediately drawn towards Him as the primary focus for all that is happening in the scene. To be truly the church, to be truly those people who live to make Christ known, all of life's changing scenes require us to cultivate this constant turning towards Christ as our primary focus. Try eradicating Christ from the central spot of this icon and the scene becomes one of passivity and ineffectiveness on behalf of the three principal disciples, and chaos and meaninglessness on behalf of the other characters, and a boy grasping at the air without hope. The moment we cast our gaze towards anything but Christ, the moment He slides out of our vision, we are left looking not just at nothing, but anything to fill the void.

Surrounding Christ's head is a halo or nimbus, which signifies the holiness of Christ. As Jesus and the Father are one, the light that flows from Jesus is the light of total intimacy. "God is light," says John in his first epistle (1 John 1: 5) and so God is made visible to humankind through Jesus by the common life that they share. The doorway that is Jesus (John 10: 7) is fully open, allowing the totality of God's life to flood the space that He occupies. And where God's life is able to emerge, where a given situation can be flooded just that little bit more, the impossible can be made possible. In Christ there are no barriers to God's possibilities. Jesus Himself makes this point to the boy's father quite explicitly in Mark's account (Mark 9: 23), and indeed the whole episode is an example of the possibilities open to God's action in and through the person of Christ. Nothing can hinder this transforming and saving love except our own degree of cooperation. We will see this being played out before us in the events of the icon in the different parties that are involved, but that is for a little later.

Above the halo are the Greek letters 'IC XC', which are Greek abbreviations for 'Jesus Christ', and as Quenot points out, "The inscription of His name confers on the icon its sacred character, its spiritual dimension" (Quenot 1991b, p. 85).

Inside the halo, although not at all clear on this icon, a cross is marked with the inscription 'O WV', the Greek letters for 'the one who is', or 'He who is'. This description points us back to the encounter that Moses had with God in Exodus 3: 14, and marks Jesus out as the one who makes known the unknowable, makes immanent the transcendent, and makes describable the one utterly indescribable. The cross on which these letters are inscribed also reminds us, particularly in the face of human struggle, human dejection and human suffering, that Jesus experiences this complete sense of hopelessness and abandonment. The face-to-face encounter of the boy and Jesus isn't just a meeting of two people; it is a meeting of God in Christ, who accommodates Himself to someone deemed to be one of the lowest forms of life by society's standards. A clue to this accommodation can be seen in the slightly stooped posture of the figure of Christ as he leans forward towards the boy. In a description of the icon *The Descent into Hell*, Solrunn Nes refers to the "divine descent". She writes:

> *The incarnation, God's visible appearance as a man, was a form of divine descent consisting of many steps. When Christ let himself be baptised, he subjected himself to the condition of sinful man. And further, by going down into the water, he let himself be covered in matter. He took still one more step down when he was buried in the depths of the earth. But by descending into Hell, Christ reached existentially, life's deepest abyss.*
>
> Nes (2004, p. 83)

In this "divine descent", Christ stoops. He gets down on the same level in a gesture of blessing and healing to the despised, rejected and ostracised, and in doing so not only indicates the beauty that lies in the heart of the other as seen by God, but offers all of us the example to do the same.

Staying with the full figure of Christ for the moment, we are given yet another set of indications as to the identity of the one whose actions display that of promise, authority and fulfilment. The clothing, consisting of a tunic (chiton), usually red in colour and worn as an undergarment, a cape (himaton) or outer garment worn over the tunic and usually blue: both are symbolic of Christ's two natures – the human and the divine. On Christ's right arm is an ornamental band (stichos), reminiscent of the Roman imperial court and indicative of high office. His right hand extends to the boy in a gesture of blessing, and in Christ's left hand is a rolled up scroll, which is a symbol of Christ's pre-existence as the Logos, or the word of God. This is God's eternal word who stands before us – the one who knows us from our mother's womb (Psalm 139: 13) and the one who promises to be with us always (Matthew 28: 20). All these features are particularly recognisable in the icon of Christ Pantocrator (The All Ruler, or He Who Rules the Universe), the judge and friend of sinners.

We gaze upon Christ the king of the universe, the supreme judge of the living and the dead. Knowing that we will all stand before Christ as judge is worth much reflection. However, the presence of Christ as judge in the icon offers some clues to the nature of this judgement and a reminder to us of where judgement and a judgemental attitude truly lie. Firstly, and this must be made quite clear, the boy is brought to Christ to be healed. There is no mention in the accounts that the boy's condition has anything to do with sin or any wrongdoing whatsoever. There is no correlation between his physical condition and past sins. (That is not to say that for some there may be a connecting link, but that isn't always the case, and it certainly isn't the case here.) So if we are to see in the figure of Christ characteristics of Christ as judge, we see a judge who stretches out His hand with compassion and understanding, and with the intention to make whole, to give life.

Secondly, once we realise this and begin to understand that there is only one judge and there will be only one judgement, our tendency to adopt this role time and time again has no place in our daily encounters and our relationships. This can be particularly problematic with people suffering with mental illness. As more and more people with mental health issues are being cared for within the community, they have become more visible to the community. Combined with the media in all its forms, we are presented with the stereotypical image of what is to be expected from people with mental illness. Given this kind of exposure it is just a short step towards judgementalism, and that is to assume a role that is not ours.

As we continue to be engaged by the figure of Christ, our eyes are naturally guided through the curve of His upper body and down His right arm, where we see Christ's extended hand in a gesture of blessing and healing. Now that we have been brought into the presence of Christ, the iconographer skilfully allows our eyes to follow the natural flow of Christ's gesture towards the object of His love and concern: the boy himself. But before we come into the presence of the boy in more detail there is time to be spent looking at the hands, particularly the possible significance of the gap between Christ's hands and the boy's.

We are aware from reading the account of the healing in Mark's gospel that the moment Christ took hold of the boy's hand, the boy was "raised up". The language here again is very revealing. Mark uses the word *egeirien*, "lifting up", which brings to mind resurrection, and this is indeed what Mark has in mind by using another resurrection verb *aneste*, "arose". The hand that we contemplate in the icon is also a doctrinal statement. The sign of the blessing, with the position of the three fingers in reference to the Trinity, reminds us that Christ does not work on His own. Through the Holy Spirit of God and with God His Father in a unity of total love, the entire life of the Godhead, is held, offered and given to the least of God's creatures.

The two fingers that are crossed remind us of Christ's humanity and divinity – a humanity that could feel the pain and isolation, the rejection and the hopelessness of all broken humanity and yet expose it to the fullness of God's healing and transforming life. As Rowan Williams puts it, "Jesus is a human being in whom God's action is at work without interruption or impediment" (Williams, Rowan (c), p. 65).

Reflecting on Christ – the second person of the Trinity, not in isolation from the Father and the Spirit in His work of ushering in the Kingdom – offers the pattern for our own working in this area of mental health. Briefly, whatever our involvement of care, friendship or activity, we do so with the support and in the company of others. These may include professional care givers such as multi-disciplinary mental health teams including psychiatry, psychology, nursing, GPs, social workers, advocates, family members, etc; and additional support from Church communities, chaplains, parishioners with some training and specialist mental health agencies. This is a theologically sound principle and of absolute priority to good practice.

So what about this gap between the blessing hand of Christ and the extended hand of the boy? We know from Mark's account that "Jesus took him by the hand", and yet the icon stops short of this moment. Could it be a reminder that despite the constant presence of God, the constant offer of acceptance, forgiveness, the eternal patient waiting and seeking for our return to Him, we are free to reject and turn away? God does not impose himself on anybody. His hand is always extended to fallen humanity. It us up to us whether we choose to reach out and grasp that hand or reject it and go it alone.

In the same way, making ourselves open and available to be used in the pastoral care of the mentally ill is something offered, never forced, and our walk with those who struggle can be accepted or rejected. Even Jesus did not force himself and could do nothing in Nazareth, where His presence was rejected (Mark 6: 1–6). The space between the hands of Christ and the boy signifies not only God's utter love of creating creatures that share in His freedom and can exercise that freedom, but it also signifies humanity's capacity to choose life or death.

THE BOY

The iconographic technique of hierarchical perspective allows the observer to locate that which is of primary importance and what is to be the attention of primary focus. In the icon before us we see that Christ dominates the scene and is therefore first in the hierarchical order. When our eyes are drawn towards the boy we see the bottom rung of the hierarchical ladder. In the composition before us the boy adopts the lowest position. This is not only significant with regard to the physical effects of his condition, it is a reflection of his importance within the group, within his culture. Within our own culture those of us who experience mental illness will observe on a regular basis this non-importance and rejection. Marion Carson puts it well when she writes:

> *... people who have mental health problems can find themselves rejected by their families, friends and the general public. They are sometimes seen as problematic ... They are often marginalised, too 'different' to be absorbed comfortably into mainstream society.*

Carson (2008b, p. XV and XVI)

The boy's size, and his position in relation to the others in the icon reflects smallness, insignificance, someone easily to be overlooked. And yet, in accordance with what was remarked upon earlier in this book about the importance of the mentally ill in relation to Christ, the boy is still the one feature in this icon that our eyes are guided towards after the person of Christ himself.

The synoptic narratives all describe the physical symptoms of the boy's torment. He is "thrown down", he suffers "convulsions" and Mark describes in greater detail the effects the boy's condition has on his physical being, and we can read this into the icon. But what the icon also shows us, which we can infer from the Gospel narratives, is something of the emotional torment that can accompany mental illness.

So many times the image of this boy comes to mind when, as a chaplain, I sit with patients in the psychiatric unit, especially those who are frightened by the voices that they hear internally or externally. Or the bewildered patient who is brought into the unit for the first time and tries to explain that they should not be there. Or the woman who pleads to be given respite from yet another descent into depression. Or the man who is distressed because the family he loves cannot cope with him being at home any more because they fear his inconsistent behaviour. The boy represents them all. The pleading outstretched arm, the disorientation reflected in the body shape, the intense look towards someone who might understand, and the easily missed hand that touches the father's foot. A touch that speaks of the longing for something familiar, for something certain, for love and acceptance, and for someone being there.

The person who meets the criterion of "someone being there" in the Gospel, and, as we shall go on to see, in the icon itself, is the boy's father. The father–son relationship is important for establishing the boy's identity as a person. Again it may seem a small point and easily overlooked, but allowing the written text and the icon to portray the boy as a person in a relationship reminds us that this is some*one* and not some *thing*. What do I mean by that? It is not uncommon for people with known mental health problems to be described as "that schizophrenic" or "that depressive" or "he is a psychotic", and within the context of the Gospel passage, "that demoniac" or "epileptic". These are labels that are frequently used to categorise a person who is immediately reduced to being some thing rather than someone.

Norman Autton gives a wonderful example that makes this point in his classic book *The Pastoral Care of the Mentally Ill*. Acknowledging several sources, he quotes:

> *Oh that we might recapture a little bit of the spirit of a St Francis, who deliberately did not see the mob for the men ... He only saw the image of God multiplied but never monotonous. To him a man was always a man and did not disappear in a dense crowd any more than in a desert ... there was never a man who looked into those brown burning eyes without being certain that Francis Bernadone was really interested in him; in his own individual life from the cradle to the grave; that he himself was being valued and taken seriously.*

> Autton (1969, p. 22)

Whatever diagnoses a person has, that person's identity as a unique man, a unique women, made in the image of God, is not absorbed or categorised by that diagnostic label. We are not dealing with just another individual who can be lumped together with other individuals who happened to have the same symptoms that warrant a 'catch all' diagnosis. Always from a Christian perspective we are with 'persons' first and foremost – persons with hopes, desires, aspirations, failures and potential. Whatever may interrupt or prevent that person's growth towards a deeper sense of personhood and relationship, we are still dealing with the flesh and blood that God chose to be part of in and through Jesus Christ, which makes all flesh and blood something to be valued.

Look again at the icon of the boy. We see the reaching out into the mystery of Christ's love, aware that somewhere within that grasp are the creator's hands waiting to recreate. And it may be that the hands that first take hold in a recreative way are the hands of God working through the hands of you and me. And then there is the direction of the boy's gaze. A gaze that longs for something knowable, tangible, something to ground him and grounds us, in our personal identity as persons because of our relationship with other persons who see beyond the brokenness to a place where God himself sees each and every one of us.

The father brings his son, not an epileptic or demoniac, and whatever the outcome, he will always be his son. How others see it will either reinforce this special bond and strengthen the environment and conditions that make for the possibilities of healing, or they will erect the barrier of pigeonholing and see what they are conditioned to see.

In many ways this reaching out in faith and the holding on to the father's foot, coupled with the intense gaze towards his father, is an echo of the father's words as reported by Mark. The father cries, "I believe; help my unbelief." What the father says in words, the son displays in his reach, his touch, his gaze.

THE FATHER OF THE BOY

The tenderness that is displayed, in word and icon, between the father and the son in many ways parallels the tenderness previously shown on the Mount of Transfiguration between God the Father and Christ the Son. On the Mount, the disciples heard from the overshadowing cloud the words, "This is my beloved Son, in whom I take delight; listen to Him" (Matthew 17: 5b). Contemplating these words as they descend from the mountain, the disciples must have surely recognised the echo of these words in the scene that confronted them, the scene we have in the icon. Here they hear the words of another father whose primary concern is his son. "Teacher, I beg you to look upon my son, for he is my only child" (Luke 9: 38b). In a similar way, too similar to ignore, the father too is saying, or wants to be able to say, "This is *my* son. Listen to *him*." Are we here able to see something of the unique relationship that Christ has, and, by association, that we should have, between himself and the mentally ill? The father of the son presents his son, and in effect says, "Listen to him, but not only him; listen to all the marginalised, the outcasts, the voiceless." For the father cares and loves his son even to the point of being able to say, "You may despise and abuse him, you may not know what to make of him, but he is my son, and with regard to me I am still well pleased." (How many parents are still able to say this out of deep affection and love for many a child categorised as 'different'?) It does not take a great leap of the imagination to see that these things are equally applicable to Christ, and equally applicable to what God the loving Father has to say about His Son.

"I believe; help my unbelief." The iconographer captures in a profound way the catalogue of experiences that have brought the father to utter these words from the depths of one in desperation. This, coupled with the words "If you can do anything ..." indicates that Christ is the only possibility left to him. The father expresses what most of us think probably a lot of the time if we are truly honest, and we will all have reasons as to why that is the case. Here I want to explore what lies behind the father's plea. However, it is important to point out that whatever brings us to this point of our faith journey (and there will be times) especially as a chaplain, a faith community or, as we shall see, a carer, it is not always the strength of our faith that allows us to approach God in a dialogue of raw honesty; it can be the poverty of our faith, something the psalmists knew all too well.

"If you can do anything ..." says the father. "Take pity on *us*." The cry from the father, and by association the family as a whole, is an extension of the suffering of the son. The raised arms of the father, and his body language, are a display of frustration, grief and exasperation. His demeanour is of one who has reached the limit for more or less the same reasons that many families and carers experience today. If we as chaplains and faith communities are living the truth of our faith as we are reminded by the icon, then the icon of the father becomes the bearer of what, as Christians, we can be mindful of amongst the carers in our parishes, congregations and, in the case of chaplains, our long-stay units. And if we are mindful of some of the problems, we may be better placed to be able to act or to be approached. So what could lie behind those raised arms of the father and his plea for help?

1. The strain of watching a loved one suffer.
2. Feelings of inadequacy and hopelessness at not being able to take the suffering away.
3. Frustration born out of the frequency of relapse and the problems that ensue.
4. The possibility of self-blame. That somehow the conditions have been created to bring the problem into existence or make the problem worse.
5. The struggle to hold family life together when the illness takes over every aspect of the household's life. Luke tells us that this is the father's only son, but for some families where there are siblings the constant attention towards the one with mental illness can and does cause family splits and estrangement.
6. Anguish at having to face the occasional bouts of hostility and non-cooperation when a loved one

begins to decline into some form of illness. This may also involve the responsibility to be the instigator of help when the loved one refuses to accept that anything is wrong.

7. Disintegration of one's own coping mechanisms.
8. Disruption of quality of life for all concerned.
9. Frustration towards those who have been set apart to offer and provide specific help, (here the group of disciples behind the father in the icon may represent those 'set apart') including the system of care provided by the psychiatric and health services, and maybe even indifferent faith communities. "I brought him to your disciples but they could not heal him" (Matthew 17: 16).

This is by no means a definitive list, and the image of the father may also express several other pertinent experiences and emotions, some of which have been experienced by many a mental health chaplain who stands in close proximity to families and carers. These can include:

1. Resentment towards the one being cared for due to the disruption to the carer's life and time consuming-nature of being the carer.
2. Embarrassment at having a 'problem' in the family.
3. The stigma associated with mental illness attached to the family and immediate carers.
4. Family ostracised by the neighbours and local

community.

5. Marginalisation by society at large.

6. Lack of support and understanding by care agencies and faith communities.

7. Faith is challenged and God's activity/inactivity is questioned (the "if you can ..." of the father in his request to Christ).

8. Anxiety and anger towards the loved one, who self-imposes isolation, removing themselves from family and friends.

These are just some indications of what families, carers and friends feel and experience when overtaken by mental illness in their midst. In the Gospel the father steps forward with his son and seeks out the help they both evidently need. For those offering help this can present a great challenge and requires knowledge of one's own capabilities, the understanding that it is not a single-handed quest and access to professional advice is all important. Some of these points will feature again when discussion turns to the two groups of disciples in the icon – the disciples behind the father and the disciples behind Christ.

Some carers are anonymous, and for whatever reason remain outside the orbit of any support available. For those who we do not see, it is imperative to create an environment, especially in our parishes, where the door is not just open, but is knowingly and by reputation to be a welcome place for any in our community who are perceived by the culture as 'different'. The Gospels repeatedly announce this; the icon shows it.

In our final look into the icon, the two groups of disciples, on the left and the right, may help us to explore our role as Christians and faith communities a little more.

THE DISCIPLES

Behind the figure of the father, our eyes almost dance between the several heads that constitute the group of disciples that are locked in a world of discussion, oblivious to what is happening right under their noses. In complete contrast, on the far left of the icon stand the disciples Peter, James and John. They are composed, attentive, watchful. Peter, who stands immediately behind Christ, (this is indeed significant, as we shall see) seems almost lost in concentration. The two groups of disciples, as well as being at both extremeties of the icon, to the left and to the right – one group before Christ, the other group behind Christ – are also on the extremes too in relation to the priority given to Christ himself.

Context is all important to these adopted positions, which becomes just as important to contemporary twenty-first-century eyes. If ever an icon could speak directly of the current gradual loss of Christian identity in the chaplaincy setting as it engages with a post-religious culture, or some of our church communities that have their gaze fixed on numbers or survival or capitulation to cultural trends, it is here in these two groups of disciples. And it is not a question of who is right or who is wrong, for both groups acknowledge Christ. It is more of a question of 'distraction', especially the distraction of 'self', wanting the self to increase in relation to Christ rather than decrease; and, of course, the multiple distractions of others around us all competing to increase.

It has to be said that there is a certain amount of sympathy to be had with these disciples behind the boy's father as they ponder their apparent failure and argue with the teachers, and all in the public gaze. It could be argued that their inability to heal the boy was as a direct result of the absence of Christ, who, with Peter, James and John, was on the Mountain of Transfiguration. However, they had already been powerful contributors to the ministry of healing in the absence of Christ (Mark 6: 13). So we have to look elsewhere for possible causes for their inability towards creating a favourable environment where the Kingdom had every opportunity to be more present. For example, Rowan Williams talks about the possibility of

> *...a really intense prayer or a really holy life can open the world up that bit more to God's purposes so that unexpected things happen ... It isn't a process we can manipulate; miracles aren't magic, and we could never have a comprehensive manual of techniques for securing what we pray for... All we know is that we are called to pray, to trust and to live with integrity before God (to live 'holy lives') in such a way as to leave the door open, to let things come together so that love can come through.*
> Williams (2007e, p. 45)

We must not be too hard on these disciples, whose position of apparent failure is one that mental health chaplains, parish clergy, all Christians will experience.

So what seems to be some of the contributing factors that may have hindered their ministry to this particular boy and his father, that are equally applicable to our own calling in this area of care?

Firstly, there is the possible pressure of engaging with an unbelieving culture; secondly, the question of humility; thirdly, and probably the most important – a lack of preparation.

In response to the father's request for his boy to be healed, and his claim that the disciples could not do it, Christ describes the gathered crowd as an "unbelieving generation" (Mark 9: 19). Was this meant for the disciples ears too? It is not certain, but the situation is familiar to that of our own day, although again to paraphrase Chesterton, "When people stop believing in God, they don't believe in nothing, they believe in anything." That "anything" falls within the parameters of 'spiritual needs' as opposed to 'religious needs'. Now it is one thing to meet those needs and even engage with them, but in doing so we need to be fairly clear of where our spiritual formation lies – in this case, the Christian faith – otherwise, at best, we have nothing unique to bring to the table. It requires a great deal of stamina, experience and indeed grace to engage with an "unbelieving generation" without being argumentative, coercive, pious or arrogant. But engage we will and that engagement begins with physical presence and the employment of language that should always endeavour to be Gospel shaped.

In the context of the Gospel narrative and the icon, the father reaches out to the disciples in the absence of Christ. He approaches them as if he were approaching Christ. This is not a bad way of describing our own role. Consideration must also be given to the effects of the crowd, the "unbelieving generation", on the disciples themselves. They obviously had some influence on the disciples, and their argument may have been persuasive, plausible, even inviting. However, the effect rendered the father's request unanswered and may even have driven the father to the point of questioning *his* faith. This may be what lies behind his cry: "I believe; help my unbelief". It is sobering to realise that our own approach, if we are not careful, may be the cause of some to question the relevance of faith after all, and too much capitulation to an "unbelieving generation" or, for the purposes of this essay, the post-religious spirituality agenda, needs a serious degree of watchfulness.

St Benedict, in Chapter 1 of the 'Rule', describes "four kinds of monks", that reflect the different approaches by some to the monasticism of his day. They are the 'cenobites', the 'anchorites', the 'sarabaites' and the 'gyrovagues'. Reflecting on these four types of monks, Esther de Waal remarks that each group can say something of our own attitudes and approaches to Christian discipleship, and in effect can be used as a "yardstick" (Waal 1995, pp. 14–17).

Of the four groups, the third group, the sarabaites, are described by Benedict in these terms:

> *... the most detestable kind of monks ... still loyal to the world by their actions ... The law is what they like to do, whatever strikes their fancy. Anything they believe in and choose they call holy, anything they dislike they consider forbidden.*
>
> Fry (1982, p. 20)

This is a fair description of the spirituality agenda today, and while it must be said that it would be pure speculation to accuse the disciples in the icon of travelling this far down the road of total assimilation to the "unbelieving generation", there might just be the hint that that is the horizon to which their attention is directed. For one disciple in the group, this may well be a present reality. Notice the person on the immediate right, who is presented to us in profile. In iconography this is not good. As Quenot makes clear:

> *In iconography, only people who have not attained holiness are seen in profile ... A profile diverts this direct contact to a certain extent and depersonalises the relation ... By their frontality, figures in the icon attract the spectator, and open to him their inner life.*
>
> Quenot (1991c, pp. 93–94)

The ideal in reference to the four kinds of monks are the cenobites, for whom Benedict wrote the 'Rule'. They are those who belong to a monastery under a rule and an abbot

(Fry, p. 20). Using Esther de Waal's approach of adopting these descriptions of the monks as a "yardstick" for contemporary discipleship, we can see that the 'monastery' for us, as disciples, is the whole world, i.e. wherever we find ourselves. The 'Rule', as it was for St Benedict, equates to the disciplines that continually point us to Christ and the making known of the Gospel, and 'the abbot' functions as a reminder to us that what we do, we do in relationship and in communion with others who have more experience and never by our own authority, which is especially important when journeying with the mental ill.

Then there is the question of humility – another pointer that may account for their failure. There are two possible clues to this. Mark tells us that the encounter with the boy and the father brought about an argument with the teachers of the law. In the section on 'Humility' in Abbot Christopher Jamison's book *Finding Sanctuary*, he writes:

> *If you examine human interactions that go wrong, whether in bitter arguments or wars, there is usually somewhere a lack of humility and an excess of arrogance.*
>
> Jamison (2006b, p. 95)

Of course that does not mean to say that they were arguing with each other, but before we place all the blame on the teachers of the law there must surely be some relation between this episode and the very next episode in the Synoptics, where the disciples are challenged over their argument about who was the greatest (Mark 9: 33–36, Luke 9: 46–50, Matthew 18: 1–4). Here Matthew places the discourse with Peter about paying the Temple Tax prior to a discussion about who the greatest will be in the Kingdom. There does seem to be a question mark over the disciples' ability to practise humility and trust totally in God and not in their own self-exaltation.

This brings us back to what was said earlier in this essay about the caring relationship. When we practise humility the danger of seeing the caring relationship as one of 'them and us': me the carer, you the cared for; me being whole, you being broken; is transformed into one of 'us and Christ' i.e. us being cared for by Christ; both broken and not broken being brought into the wholeness of Christ.

Underscoring all this, of course, and potentially something that the disciples failed to appreciate, is the importance of preparation. Matthew gives us the fullest indication of this possibility with the addition of the discipline of "fasting" to "prayer" as the means to deal with this given situation (Matthew 17: 21).

It is not implausible to suggest that the disciples, in the absence of Christ, failed to continue and practise quiet times set apart for the purpose of orientating their thoughts and passions towards God. A bishop, very experienced in the healing and deliverance ministry, once said to a group of us, "Ensure you are faithful to your calling, say the daily office, go to the Eucharist as often as you can, confess your sins, and read the Scriptures. This is the platform from which all pastoral work should be undertaken." The point is well made for it allows our presence, our words and actions to be formed and informed by the close presence of God, in whose company we are not strangers.

In contrast to this group of disciples behind the father, we have the three disciples – Peter, James and John – on the left of the icon, directly behind Christ. There is no telling if they would have been any more successful in healing the boy if they had remained with the other disciples in the absence of Christ. However, what their position in the icon does show us, what we are drawn into, is the strongest statement that defines every pastoral encounter, the lens through which ministry is truly Christocentric.

First, the context. Prior to the encounter with the boy and his father, Peter, in a moment of inspiration and revelation at Caesarea Philippi, gives voice to the realisation that Jesus is the Christ (Matthew 16: 13ff, Mark 8: 27ff, Luke 9: 18ff) and this is fully endorsed when Peter, James and John witness Christ Transfigured (notice the mountain rising up in the icon linking the two episodes), but not before Peter is rebuked by Christ for misunderstanding the path that He has to take: one of humiliation and death.

The rebuke is well known. Christ says to Peter, "Get behind me, Satan." To understand the ways of God, to follow, to learn, to "decrease", we must acknowledge that Christ goes *before* us. And then again on the Mount of Transfiguration a cloud descends on the disciples and a voice utters the words, "This is my son whom I love, listen to him." With these incidents in mind, look again at these disciples in the icon. Peter stands with James and John *behind* Christ, and his attentiveness is evidence enough that here is a man who is listening. Follow and listen. Mother Teresa brought this to the attention of one of her sisters. This is what she said:

> *As for me – thank God we have been told to follow Christ. As I have not to go ahead of Him, even in the darkness the path is sure ... There was no need to 'find the way' but rather to 'follow the way' that Jesus had already walked. This conviction she transmitted to her sisters. Once I saw a sister with a long face going out for Apostolate, so I called her to my room and I asked her, "What did Jesus say, to carry the Cross in front of Him or to follow Him?" With a big smile she looked at me and said, "To follow Him." So I asked her, "Why are you trying to go ahead of Him?" She left my room smiling. She had understood the meaning of following Jesus.*
>
> Kolodiejchuk (2007, p. 221)

And so we have come back full circle. Following Christ, placing Christ before us, both in the actions we take towards a people who are seen by society as the last taboo, and seeing Him in those same people whose image we are all made.

The icon uniquely exists as a gateway, a window, a door, that place where the Kingdom floods in and we see with our eyes, and are seen by the eyes of the one who calls us all to be living icons.

In the words of the hymn by H.D. Rawnsley, written for those who are partners with Christ in the healing ministry, be it chaplain or faith community:

> *Before them set thy holy will,*
> *That they with heart and soul*
> *To thee may consecrate their skill*
> *And make the sufferer whole.*

The Healing of the Demon Possessed Boy in the Synoptic Gospels

MATTHEW 17: 14–21

14 And when they came to the crowd, a man came up to him and kneeling before him said, *15* "Lord, have mercy on my son, for he is an epileptic and he suffers terribly; for often he falls into the fire, and often into the water. *16* And I brought him to your disciples, and they could not heal him." *17* And Jesus answered, "O faithless and perverse generation, how long am I to be with you? How long am I to bear with you? Bring him here to me." *18* And Jesus rebuked him, and the demon came out of him, and the boy was cured instantly. *19* Then the disciples came to Jesus privately and said, "Why could we not cast it out?" *20* He said to them, "Because of your little faith. For truly, I say to you, if you have faith as a grain of mustard seed, you will say to this mountain, 'Move from here to there,' and it will move; and nothing will be impossible for you."*

*Other ancient authorities insert verse *21*: "But this kind never comes out except by prayer and fasting."

MARK 9: 14–29

14 And when they came to the disciples, they saw a great crowd about them, and scribes arguing with them. *15* And immediately all the crowd, when they saw him, were greatly amazed, and ran up to him and greeted him. *16* And he asked them, "What are you discussing with them?" *17* And one of the crowd answered him, "Teacher, I brought my son to you, for he has a dumb spirit; *18* and wherever it seizes him, it dashes him down; and he foams and grinds his teeth and becomes rigid; and I asked your disciples to cast it out, and they were not able." *19* And he answered them, "O, faithless generation, how long am I to be with you? How long am I to bear with you? Bring him to me." *20* And they brought the boy to him; and when the spirit saw him, immediately it convulsed the boy, and he fell on the ground and rolled about, foaming at the mouth. *21* And Jesus asked his father, "How long has he had this?" And he said, "From childhood. *22* And it has often cast him into the fire and into the water, to destroy him; but if you can do anything, have pity on us and help us." *23* And Jesus said to him, "If you can! All things are possible to him who believes." *24* Immediately the father of the child cried out and said, "I believe; help my unbelief!" *25* And when Jesus saw that a crowd came running together, he rebuked the unclean spirit, saying to it, "You dumb and deaf spirit, I command you, come out of him, and never enter him again." *26* And after crying out and convulsing him terribly, it came out, and the boy was like a corpse; so that most of them said, "He is dead." *27* But Jesus took him by the hand and lifted him up, and he arose. *28* And when he had entered the house, his disciples asked him privately, "Why could not we cast it out?" *29* And he said to them, "This kind cannot be driven out by anything but prayer."*

*Other ancient authorities add "and fasting".

Luke 9: 37–43

*37*On the next day, when they had come down from the mountain, a great crowd met him. *38*And behold, a man from the crowd cried, "Teacher, I beg you to look upon my son, for he is my only child; *39*and behold, a spirit seizes him, and he suddenly cries out; it convulses him till he foams, and shatters him, and will hardly leave him. *40*And I begged your disciples to cast it out, but they could not." *41*Jesus answered, "O, faithless and perverse generation, how long am I to be with you and bear with you? Bring your son here." *42*While he was coming, the demon tore him and convulsed him. But Jesus rebuked the unclean spirit, and healed the boy, and gave him back to his father. *43*And all were astonished at the majesty of God.

Taken from *The Revised Standard Version Common Bible.*

Appendix

My friend thinks he is demonically oppressed, but his vicar tells him that's impossible. What should I advise him to do?

Evil spirits figure prominently in the healing narratives of the New Testament (e.g. Mark 1: 21–28; 32–34; 3: 10–12), but today many Christians would argue that symptoms which were then attributed to evil spirits would now be treated as having a psychological cause and dealt with by drugs, psychiatry, counselling, etc.

Some of them would go further and claim that the biblical references to the devil and his minions can be dismissed as examples of how a primitive society tried to explain the problem of evil by ascribing it to malevolent spiritual forces outside human control. Consequently the gospels, written in the first century AD, speak of Jesus Christ's authority over these spiritual forces. This was the religious and cultural milieu into which Jesus was born and which he accepted as a human being of that era. People sharing this point of view regard the concept of a spiritual warfare, so deeply embedded in the Christian teaching, as a hangover from this, enshrined in the Bible. They urge us to abandon such outdated concepts and recognise that, if we knew all the evidence, everything that is evil can be traced ultimately to natural causes. For them, therefore, there is no such thing as being 'demonically oppressed'.

This view is not accepted by other Christians. Even those who do not accept the New Testament understanding of healings as just outlined still believe that Jesus's teaching on evil and his personal spiritual battle against Satan cannot be explained away just to satisfy the assumptions of a science-dominated world view. Jesus included in the Lord's Prayer the words, 'Deliver us from evil', and in the experience of millions of his followers over the centuries the spiritual battle is very real indeed. Not all evil can be attributed to personal upbringing, psychological make-up, genetic programming, social pressures or other natural causes. For these Christians the words 'Satan', 'the devil' and 'demons' may have a primitive mythological flavour about them. However, they represent the reality of evil influences which affect the lives of people to varying degrees – influences which often seem so mysteriously aimed at particular individuals, families, groups and nations that the adjective 'personal' as appropriate in describing them (e.g. in the phrase 'a personal devil'). The appropriate ministry for people troubled by such evil influences is prayer for deliverance or formal exorcism in acute cases. We have discussed these ministries in Chapter 9.

Your friend should be advised that it is extremely unusual for anyone to recognise demonic oppression in themselves and that he should first seek the advice of his medical practitioner, who may suggest counselling or perhaps psychiatric treatment. However, if he follows the doctor's advice for a while and is still troubled, he should seek spiritual help. Then, if the vicar (for whatever reason) is unable or unwilling to minister to him, he should ask the vicar if he can make an appointment to see the bishop's advisor for the healing ministry, or write to the bishop himself.

Extract from: The Archbishops' Council 2000 *A Time to Heal: A Contribution Towards the Ministry of Healing*, pp. 230–231 (Church House Publishing)

References

The Archbishops' Council (2000), *A Time to Heal: A Contribution Towards the Ministry of Healing*, Chapter 9, p. 167 'Deliverance from Evil' (Church House Publishing)

Autton, Norman (1969), *The Pastoral Care of the Mentally Ill*, p. 22 (SPCK)

Bigham, Steven (Fr) (1998), *Heroes of the Icon*, p. 44 (Oakwood Publ.)

Ibid, p. 45

Brown, Peter (Jan 1973), 'A Dark Age Crisis: Aspects of the Iconoclastic Controversy', *The English Historical Review* Vol. 88, no. 346, pp. 5–6 (Oxford University Press)

Carson, Marion L.S. (2008a), *The Pastoral Care of People with Mental Health Problems*, p. 7 (SPCK)

Carson, Marion L.S. (2008b), *The Pastoral Care of People with Mental Health Problems*, pp. XV and XVI (SPCK)

Clark, Carlton (Dr) and Shaffer Frank (2009), *Special Moments in Orthodoxy: Icons and Their Meaning* (Orthodox Christian Network)

Crow, Gillian (2008), *Orthodoxy for Today*, p.97 (SPCK)

Fry, Timothy OSB (1982), *The Rule of St. Benedict in English* p. 20 (The Liturgical Press)

Harries, Richard and Mayr-Harting, Henry (2001a), *Christianity: Two Thousand Years*, Chapter 4 'Eastern Christianity' (Oxford University Press)

Ibid (2001b), p. 92

Hart, Aiden (2000a), *Icons and the Human Person*, p. 1 www.aidenharticons.com

Hart, Aiden (2000b), *The Icon and Pastoral Care*, p. 1 www.aidenharticons.com

Ibid (2000c), p. 5

Ibid (2000d), p. 4

Jamison, Christopher (Abbot) (2006a), *Finding Sanctuary: Monastic Steps for Everyday Life*, p. 167 (Weidenfeld and Nicolson)

Jamison, Christopher (Abbot) (2006b), *Finding Sanctuary: Monastic Steps for Everyday Life*, p. 95 (Weidenfeld and Nicolson)

Kolodiejchuk, Brian M.C. (2007), *Mother Teresa, Come Be My Light*, p. 221 (Doubleday Publ.)

Lewis, Edward (Nov 2005), 'The Last Shall Be First', *The Pastoral Review* Vol. 1,

No. 6, p. 40

Mason, Paul (Fr) (2006), Catholic NHS Chaplaincy, 'I Love You But ...' *JHCC* Vol. 7, No. 1, p. 66

Nes, Solrunn (2004), *The Mystical Language of Icons*, p. 83 (Canterbury Press)

Meeting the Religious and Spiritual Needs of Patients and Staff. Guidelines for Managers and Those involved in the Provision of Chaplaincy Spiritual and Religious Care, p. 5, NHS Guidance Document (2003) (NHS Chaplaincy)

Nolland, John (2005), The New International Greek Testament Commentary, *The Gospel of Matthew*, p.711, (Grand Rapids Michigan, W.B. Eerdmans Pub. Co. Bletchley Paternoster Press)

Pattison, Stephen (2009), 'The Challenge of Chaplaincy for Faith Communities and Scholars' – lecture given at the Cardiff School of Religious and Theological Studies.

Quenot, Michel (1991a), *The Icon: Window on the Kingdom*, p. 119 (Mowbray)

Quenot, Michel (1991b), *The Icon: Window on the Kingdom*, p. 85 (Mowbray)

Quenot, Michel (1991c), *The Icon: Window on the Kingdom*, pp. 93–94 (Mowbray)

Radcliffe, Timothy OP (2005), *What Is the Point in Being a Christian?* p. 42 (Continuum)

Schneider, Sandra M. IHM (Feb 2000a), *Religion and Spirituality: Strangers, Rivals, or Partners?* Santa Clara Lecture, Santa Clara University, Vol. 6, No. 2, pp. 11–12

Schneider, Sandra M. IHM (Feb 2000b), *Religion and Spirituality: Strangers, Rivals, or Partners?* – Santa Clara Lecture, Santa Clara University, Vol. 6, No. 2, p. 18

Swinton, John (2001), *Spirituality and Mental Health Care*, p. 11 (Jessica Kingsley Publ.)

Temple, Richard (1982), *Icons: A Search for Inner Meaning*, p. 10 (The Temple Gallery)

Waal, Esther de (1995), *A Life Giving Way: A Commentary on the Rule of St. Benedict*, Chapter 1, pp. 14–17 (Continuum)

Ware, Timothy (1997), *The Orthodox Church*, p. 33 (Penguin Books)

Williams, Jane (Nov 2007), *Sixth Norman Autton Lecture, Lambeth Palace London*, p. 5

Williams, Rowan (May 2007a), *Christianity: Public Religion and the Common Good*, Archbishop of Canterbury Lecture, p. 5 www.archbishopofcanterbury.org

Williams, Rowan (May 2007b), *Christianity: Public Religion and the Common Good*, Archbishop of Canterbury Lecture, p. 4 www.archbishopofcanterbury.org

Williams, Rowan (2007c), *Tokens of Trust*, p. 143 (Canterbury Press)

Williams, Rowan (2007d), *Tokens of Trust*, p. 65 (Canterbury Press)

Williams, Rowan (2007e), *Tokens of Trust*, p. 45 (Canterbury Press)

Wright, Tom (Bishop) (Summer 2005), 'The Christian Challenge in the Post-Modern World', *Response* (Seattle Pacific University Magazine) Vol. 28, No. 2